COMPLETE GUIDE TO BUNION SURGERY

Essential Handbook For Expert Techniques, Recovery Tips, And Pain Management For Optimal Foot Health

DR. BRUNO HORAN

Copyright © 2023 by Dr. Bruno Horan

All rights reserved. Except for brief quotations embodied in critical reviews and certain other noncommercial uses permitted by copyright law, no part of this publication may be reproduced, distributed, or transmitted in any form or by any means, Including photocopying, recording, or other electronic or mechanical methods, without the prior written permission of the publisher.

Disclaimer:

The information provided in this book, is intended for general informational purposes only and should not be considered as professional advice.

The author has made every effort to ensure the accuracy of the information presented. However, readers are advised to consult with a qualified healthcare professional before attempting any herbal remedies or making significant changes to their wellness routine. Individual health conditions vary, and what may be suitable for one person may not be appropriate for another.

It is important to note that the author is not in any endorsement deal, partnership, or affiliation with any organization, brand, or company mentioned in this book. Any references to specific products or services are based on the author's personal experience or general knowledge and do not imply an endorsement or promotion of those products or services

Contents

CHAPTER ONE 17
SELECTING A SURGERY 17
When To Get Surgical Treatment For Bunions 17

Different Bunion Surgery Types........................18

Advantages And Drawbacks Of Bunion Surgery ..18

Speaking With An Orthopedic Surgeon Or Podiatrist...19

Changes In Pre-Surgery Lifestyle.......................19

CHAPTER TWO 21
PRE-OPINION SETTLEMENT 21
Comprehensive Medical Assessments..................21

Getting Your House Ready For Rehab................22

What To Bring To The Medical Facility 23

Exercises And Conditioning Before Surgery 24

CHAPTER THREE 27
THE OPERATIONAL METHODS..........................27
An Extensive Overview Of Typical Bunion Procedures 27

Traditional Surgery Vs. Minimally Invasive Surgery 29

What Takes Place Throughout The Procedure 29

Anesthesia's Function In Bunion Surgery............30

Frequently Used Surgical Instruments.................31

CHAPTER FOUR 35

IMMEDIATE CARE AFTER OPERATION 35

Anticipations For The Rehab Room 35

Medications And Pain Management....................36

Initial At-Home Postoperative Care 36

Initial Consultation With Your Surgeon...............37

CHAPTER FIVE 39

PERMANENT RECOVERY...39

A Schedule For Recovery And Milestones 41

The Value Of Confirmation Meetings...................43

Exercises For Physical Therapy And Rehabilitation 45

Modifying Everyday Tasks While Recovering.......48

Keeping Bunions From Recurring........................50

CHAPTER SIX...53

COMMON ISSUES AND DIFFICULTIES 53

Handling Pain And Discomfort After Surgery.......54

Handling Bruises And Swelling 55

Preventing Infections And Recognizing Warning Signs..56

Taking Care Of Cosmetic Concerns And Scarring 57

Taking Care Of Nerve Damage And Mobility Problems 58

CHAPTER SEVEN 60

COMMONLY ASKED QUESTIONS OR FAQS............60

How Likely Is It That Bunions Will Recur? 60

How Soon After Surgery Can I Go On Foot? 61

Will I Require Certain Shoes After My Surgery? ..61

Can I Lose My Ability To Exercise After Bunion Surgery?..62

What Kind Of Lifestyle Adjustments Are Required After Surgery? 63

CONCERNING THIS BOOK

"Bunion Surgery" is a thorough handbook that offers persons coping with the discomfort and difficulties caused by bunions a beacon of knowledge and support. It is more than just a book. This book expertly and sympathetically navigates every facet of the bunion journey, from its thorough examination of the anatomy of the condition to the complexities of post-operative care.

The basic knowledge about bunions, including their definition, symptoms, and underlying causes, is provided to readers at the beginning of the book. With this fundamental understanding, people are better equipped to identify and treat their disease early on and make well-informed decisions regarding their course of treatment.

The book's in-depth analysis of the surgical path is one of its best qualities. It gives readers the tools to make this crucial decision with clarity and confidence by exploring the many kinds of bunion procedures, balancing the advantages over the disadvantages, and offering insights into the consultation process with medical professionals.

Beyond just preparing, "Bunion Surgery" takes readers step-by-step through the entire surgical process, from psychological preparation and pre-surgery assessments to the specifics of the surgical techniques. Through its direct approach to frequent issues and problems, the book acts as a comforting guide, demystifying the procedure and providing helpful tips for a quicker recovery.

Most importantly, adding a human touch through real-life success stories and testimonials gives readers hope and motivation for when they start their recovery journeys. Furthermore, the FAQ section answers frequently asked questions and clear up misconceptions, enhancing the book's reputation as a reliable guide for anybody navigating the complications of bunion surgery.

Essentially, "Bunion Surgery" becomes more than just an educational tool—rather, it becomes a lifeline for those who are looking for direction, comfort, and certainty as they proceed toward relief and healing. This book is a vital resource for anyone dealing with bunions and the possibility of surgery because of its thorough covering, sympathetic writing style, and abundance of useful advice.

Overview of Bunions

Bunions, also known as hallux valgus in medical terminology, are bony protrusions that develop on the big toe joint. They frequently occur gradually, resulting in pain and suffering as the big toe bends inward toward the second toe. Even though bunions might seem like a little problem, if they are not addressed, they can have a major negative impact on quality of life and mobility.

Anatomy and Definition of a Bunion

Let's examine the anatomy of bunions to gain a better understanding of them. The metatarsophalangeal (MTP) joint is located at the base of the big toe. When the bone or tissue at this joint shifts, the big toe angles inward, leading to the formation of a bunion. The prominent hump on the side of the foot results from this mismatch. The bunion may become inflamed with time and cause pain and discomfort, particularly when walking or wearing shoes.

Signs and Symptoms to Watch Out for

Early diagnosis and treatment of bunions might be facilitated by early symptom recognition. Typical indications of a bunion are:

Bulging bump: One of the main indicators of a bunion is a prominent bulge at the base of the big toe.

Misaligned toes: When the big toe leans toward the second toe, it might crowd or overlap the other toes.

Pain and Soreness: Bunions can be painful and sore, especially when you wear shoes or exercise.

Redness and swelling: Because of the inflammation, the afflicted area may look red and swollen.

Limited mobility: Bunions can impede big toe mobility, making it challenging to walk or do specific activities.

Reasons and Involving Elements

Bunions can arise as a result of various factors, such as:

Genetics: Bunions tend to run in families, suggesting a genetic susceptibility to the disorder.

Foot structure: Bunions can be more likely to develop in those with flat feet or low arches.

Unsuitable footwear: By applying pressure to the toes and forefoot, high heels, or narrow, tight shoes can worsen bunions.

Injuries: Foot trauma or injury can cause the MTP joint to become misaligned, which can lead to a bunion.

Medical conditions: By altering the structure and functionality of the foot joints, certain illnesses, such as arthritis, can hasten the development of bunions.

How Medical Professionals Diagnose Bunions

Bunion diagnosis usually entails a thorough examination by a medical specialist, such as an orthopedic surgeon or podiatrist. As part of the assessment, the medical professional will:

Medical history: The patient's medical history, including any family history of bunions or similar foot disorders, will be enquired about by the doctor.

Physical examination: To determine the extent of the bunion, its effect on foot function, and any related symptoms, a comprehensive physical examination of the foot will be performed.

Imaging tests: To acquire precise images of the foot anatomy, X-rays may be requested. This will enable the medical professional to determine the extent of the bunion and formulate a treatment strategy.

Typical Non-Surgical Care

Bunions can frequently be treated conservatively with non-surgical methods. Typical therapy alternatives include the following:

Modifications to footwear: Wearing roomy, broad shoes helps relieve pressure on the bunion and lessen discomfort.

Orthotic devices: Personalized arch supports or orthotic inserts can help realign the foot, reduce bunion pressure, and enhance general foot function.

Protective padding and taping: By cushioning the area and lowering friction, applying protective padding or tape to the bunion helps relieve symptoms.

Medication: Ibuprofen or acetaminophen, two over-the-counter pain medicines, can help reduce the discomfort and inflammation brought on by bunions.

Physical therapy: A physical therapist's recommended targeted exercises and stretching methods will help strengthen and increase the flexibility of the foot's muscles, which will enhance its alignment and function.

People may manage their bunions and reduce discomfort by being proactive and learning about the condition's causes, symptoms, and available treatments.

While mild to moderate bunions can be relieved with non-surgical treatments, more severe cases could necessitate surgery to rectify the underlying structural deformity and return function to the foot.

Seeking advice from a healthcare expert is crucial for accurate diagnosis and customized treatment plans catered to each patient's needs.

CHAPTER ONE

SELECTING A SURGERY

It's critical to consider several variables while thinking about bunion surgery to make an informed choice. Bunions can impair your quality of life by causing pain, discomfort, and decreased movement.

Surgery may be a viable choice if conservative measures like as using orthotics, wearing appropriate footwear, and using painkillers haven't been enough to relieve the condition.

When To Get Surgical Treatment For Bunions

When non-surgical measures fail to relieve persistent discomfort, provide difficulties walking, or impede everyday activities, surgery becomes a viable option. Additionally, surgical treatment may be required if the bunion is getting worse over time or causing problems like bursitis or hammertoe.

Different Bunion Surgery Types

Bunion correction can be achieved by a variety of surgical techniques, each designed to treat different features of the deformity and meet the needs of the patient. Typical forms include arthrodesis, which entails fusing the injured joint, and osteotomy, in which the surgeon slices and realigns the bone. Exostectomy is another procedure that aims to remove the bony protrusion without displacing the joint.

Advantages And Drawbacks Of Bunion Surgery

Potential advantages of bunion surgery include pain reduction, better foot function, and improved attractiveness. Surgery can help stop further progression and lower the risk of related problems by addressing the underlying abnormality. Like every surgical operation, there are risks associated with this one as well, including infection, nerve injury, stiffness, and bunion recurrence. Making an informed choice depends on your understanding of these risks and having a conversation about them with your physician.

Speaking With An Orthopedic Surgeon Or Podiatrist

It's crucial to speak with a skilled podiatrist or orthopedic surgeon who specializes in treating foot and ankle issues before having bunion surgery. To evaluate the severity of the bunion and identify the best course of therapy, the surgeon will review your medical history, do a physical examination, and maybe request imaging tests such as X-rays during the consultation.

You will have the chance to voice your concerns, ask questions, and gain an understanding of the surgical procedure and anticipated results at this consultation.

Changes In Pre-Surgery Lifestyle

Making specific lifestyle adjustments in advance of bunion surgery can help to maximize the surgical result and speed up recovery. These modifications could be changing your footwear to fit bandages and swelling after surgery, eating a nutritious diet to promote recovery, and, if necessary, giving up smoking to lower the chance of problems. In addition, before surgery, your surgeon can suggest certain exercises or physical therapy to strengthen the foot muscles and increase the range of motion. Following these pre-surgery guidelines will help you heal more quickly and have a better result.

CHAPTER TWO

PRE-OPINION SETTLEMENT

To guarantee a smooth and satisfactory outcome, extensive pre-surgical preparation is required before undergoing bunion surgery. Pre-surgery exercises, home recovery readiness, essential hospital goods, thorough medical examinations, and psychological preparation to create reasonable expectations are all included in this preparation.

Comprehensive Medical Assessments

A vital part of getting ready for bunion surgery is going through extensive medical evaluations. Your orthopedic surgeon will usually perform a thorough examination as part of these assessments, and they may involve X-rays or other imaging tests to determine the extent of your bunion and any related deformities. To make sure you are in the best possible health for surgery, your surgeon will also go over your medical history and current prescriptions.

Your surgeon will go over the surgical alternatives that are open to you, along with the possible risks and advantages of each technique, based on the findings of these assessments.

You get the chance to voice any queries you may have and any worries you may have regarding the process during this conversation.

Getting Your House Ready For Rehab

It's essential to have your house ready for post-surgery rehabilitation if you want the healing process to be secure and comfortable.

If you live in a multi-story home, this may entail adjusting your living environment to fit your limited mobility. For example, you may need to remove any trip hazards like loose carpets or electrical cords and establish a recuperation room on the bottom floor.

During your recuperation, you might also need to make plans to help with everyday duties like cooking, cleaning, and transportation.

Establishing a support network helps facilitate the discharge process from the hospital and facilitates a more seamless recuperation.

What To Bring To The Medical Facility

To guarantee your comfort and convenience throughout your stay, you must bring any necessary goods to the hospital on the day of your surgery.

To pass the time while recovering, this may contain personal necessities like toiletries, cozy clothing, and entertainment like books or electronic gadgets.

Along with a list of your allergies and medical conditions, you should also bring any current drugs you are taking for the hospital staff to know. Remember to bring your insurance information as well as any necessary documents or consent forms that the surgeon may have given you.

Exercises And Conditioning Before Surgery

Your physician can suggest particular workouts or conditioning methods to help strengthen the muscles around your foot and increase flexibility before bunion surgery. These exercises are intended to maximize your surgical outcome and reduce the possibility of post-operative problems like weakness or stiffness.

You might receive a customized workout regimen from your physical therapist or surgeon, based on your unique requirements and capabilities. It is imperative that you attentively adhere to these instructions and share any challenges or worries you may have while undergoing pre-surgery conditioning.

Psychological Readiness and Establishing Goals

Being a major emotional and psychological experience, having bunion surgery can be difficult, therefore it's important to mentally prepare oneself for what lies ahead. This can entail being honest with your surgeon or a mental health specialist about any worries or fears you may have regarding the procedure.

Remaining upbeat and controlling expectations also need setting reasonable expectations for the surgical result and the healing process. Although bunion surgery can significantly reduce pain and enhance the appearance of your foot, it's important to realize that recovery may take some time and that your activities may be restricted during the first healing phase.

You can face bunion surgery with confidence and peace of mind, knowing that you have taken proactive actions to maximize your surgical outcome and promote a successful recovery, by addressing both the physical and psychological components of pre-surgery preparation.

26

CHAPTER THREE

THE OPERATIONAL METHODS

The term "bunion surgery," or "bunionectomy," refers to a group of surgical techniques used to treat big toe joint deformities.

These operations are usually advised for those who have a bunion and are in constant pain, have trouble walking, or have restricted mobility.

An Extensive Overview Of Typical Bunion Procedures

There are numerous popular bunion operations available, each designed to treat a distinct element of the deformity. The most common methods consist of:

Osteotomy: This corrective procedure entails repositioning the big toe by cutting and realigning its bones. To relieve strain on the joint, surgeons could remove or relocate a part of the bone.

Exostectomy: The bony protrusion (bunion) from the side of the big toe joint is removed by the surgeon during this treatment. It can ease pain and suffering from the bunion pressing on shoes, but it doesn't treat the underlying imbalance.

Arthrodesis: Also referred to as fusion surgery, arthrodesis entails joining the big toe joint's bones. Because it limits joint movement, this technique is often saved for severe instances where other methods have failed.

Resection Arthroplasty: To reduce discomfort and enhance joint function, a piece of the injured joint surface is removed. For older patients or those with severe joint injury, it is frequently advised.

The choice of technique relies on the severity of the bunion and the specific demands of the patient. Each of these surgeries has advantages and disadvantages of its own.

Traditional Surgery Vs. Minimally Invasive Surgery

Minimally invasive methods have become more and more common in bunion surgery in recent years. Compared to open surgery, these methods need fewer incisions and less tissue damage. Less scarring, quicker healing, and less postoperative pain are common outcomes of minimally invasive surgeries.

On the other hand, deeper incisions and more extensive bone cutting or realignment are usually used in traditional bunion surgery. Traditional surgery often involves more postoperative discomfort and a longer recovery period, while it may be necessary for severe instances or specific types of abnormalities.

What Takes Place Throughout The Procedure

Depending on the particular operation and the patient's choices, the patient is usually placed under either local or general anesthesia during bunion surgery. After the anesthesia wears off, the surgeon makes an incision across the bunion to gain access to the soft tissues and underlying bones.

The surgeon may realign the big toe's bones, remove extra bone, or take other remedial action to treat the deformity, depending on the method that is selected. With the least amount of harm to the surrounding structures, the bones and tissues are carefully manipulated using specialized equipment.

After making the required adjustments, the incision is sutured shut and the surgical site is covered with a bandage or dressing. Temporary plates, screws, or pins may occasionally be utilized to stabilize the bones during the early stages of recovery.

Anesthesia's Function In Bunion Surgery

During bunion surgery, anesthesia is essential to the patient's comfort and security. Local anesthetic numbs the surgical site and prevents pain signals from entering the brain. It is usually injected. This makes the surgery less uncomfortable for the patient while enabling them to stay awake and conscious.

On the other hand, general anesthesia causes unconsciousness, so the patient doesn't even know they're having surgery. To ensure the patient's comfort and safety while allowing the surgeon to work uninterrupted, it is frequently chosen for more involved or drawn-out surgeries.

The complexity of the procedure, the patient's medical history, and the surgeon's preference all play a role in the anesthetic choice. To choose the best anesthesia strategy for their particular circumstances, patients should talk over their options with their healthcare provider.

Frequently Used Surgical Instruments

A range of specialist tools are needed for bunion surgery to make the required repairs safely and efficiently. Among the tools that are most frequently used are:

Osteotomes: During osteotomy treatments, bone is sliced and shaped using these sharp, chisel-like devices.

A bone saw is a specialized saw that is used to cut bone. It is commonly used in bunion surgery to remove extra bone or make accurate cuts.

medical scissors: Designed to meet a range of medical requirements, surgical scissors are used to cut soft tissues like ligaments, tendons, and skin. They are available in different sizes and shapes.

Forceps: Throughout the process, these grabbing tools are utilized to hold and work with tissues, bones, or other surgical materials.

Surgical drills: Available in a range of sizes and configurations to suit diverse surgical requirements, surgical drills are used to drill holes in bone for the insertion of screws, pins, or other fixation devices.

Retractors: The surgeon can see more clearly and have easier access to the surgical site by using these instruments to hold tissues or organs out of the way.

Surgeons can execute bunion surgery safely and effectively with these sophisticated devices, giving their patients the best possible results.

CHAPTER FOUR

IMMEDIATE CARE AFTER OPERATION

Following your bunion surgery, you'll be brought to the recovery area, where medical staff will keep a close eye on your progress.

Anticipate a foggy feeling as the anesthesia wears off. You'll probably have a cast or surgical boot on your foot, and it will probably be bandaged.

Anticipations For The Rehab Room

Nurses will check on you in the recovery room, taking your vital signs and making sure you're comfortable. If pain management is required, they could administer cold packs to lessen swelling.

At first, you could feel a little queasy or confused, but as you relax, these feelings should go away.

Medications And Pain Management

Pain control is essential while the body heals. Painkillers will be prescribed by your surgeon to help with discomfort management. To keep ahead of the pain, you must take these drugs as prescribed. Moreover, applying cold packs and raising your foot can assist lessen pain and swelling.

Initial At-Home Postoperative Care

You will need to take care of your foot at home after being released from the hospital. Observe the guidelines provided by your surgeon on wound maintenance, medication regimen, and activity restrictions.

Unless otherwise advised, keep your foot as elevated as possible to minimize swelling and refrain from placing weight on it.

Signs of Difficulties to Be Aware of

Even though complications following bunion surgery are uncommon, it's important to watch out for any warning indications. Keep an eye out for any unusual bleeding, swelling, or discharge from the wound. Additionally, get in touch with your surgeon right away if you have excruciating pain, tingling, or numbness in your foot.

Initial Consultation With Your Surgeon

Usually, your surgeon will schedule your first follow-up appointment for you within a week or two following the procedure. Your surgeon will check your foot, take out any sutures or bandages, and monitor the status of your recovery during this visit. You have the chance to ask any questions you may have concerning your rehabilitation process during this visit. To encourage the best possible healing, make sure you adhere to any further advice your surgeon may have given you.

CHAPTER FIVE
PERMANENT RECOVERY

Beginning with bunion surgery, a path toward complete recovery and regained mobility begins. Although the actual treatment is a major step toward pain relief and deformity correction, the real change happens in the long-term recovery phase. To achieve the best outcomes during this time, patience, dedication, and following medical advice are required.

It's normal to feel some soreness, edema, and limited movement in the area surrounding the surgery site in the early stages of recuperation. But as the days go by, these symptoms progressively go away and are replaced with increased usefulness and comfort. It's critical to carefully adhere to post-operative instructions, which include elevating the foot, using ice packs, and taking prescription pain and inflammation relievers.

You'll notice gradual gains in your foot's capacity to support your weight as the weeks go by. Restorative physical therapy and mild exercises are essential for regaining range of motion, flexibility, and strength. Your doctor will create a personalized rehabilitation program for you that includes exercises to strengthen the ligaments and muscles that surround your big toe joint.

Patience is your best ally as you move from the acute to the long-term stages of healing. Although it's reasonable to want to get back to your regular activities as soon as possible, pushing yourself too hard or too soon can hinder your recovery and raise the possibility of complications. Under the supervision of your healthcare practitioner, gradually raise your exercise levels while paying attention to your body and respecting its restrictions.

It's critical to stay in constant communication with your healthcare team during the long-term rehabilitation process. To make sure you stay on course for a favorable conclusion, you should swiftly address any worries, unexpected symptoms, or queries that come up. Recovering from an illness does not always go in a straight line; there may be ups and downs. For the greatest outcomes, have faith in the knowledge of your medical specialists and adhere to the recommended treatment plan.

A Schedule For Recovery And Milestones

It's crucial to comprehend the healing process's timeframe and the benchmarks you should aim for to control expectations and maintain motivation while recovering. Although each person's journey is different, there are broad principles that might assist you in assessing your development and foreseeing significant turning points.

After bunion surgery, the main goals are to control discomfort, minimize swelling, and give the operative site time to heal. To move about safely during the first few days, you might need to use a walker or crutches, and it's usually advised to avoid putting any weight on the operated foot.

You'll probably make a follow-up appointment with your doctor within the first two weeks to discuss any concerns and have any stitches or dressings taken off. At this point, to support the foot and promote recovery, you could switch to using a splint or protective boot.

Your pain and mobility should significantly improve by the four to six-week point. During this time, many people can progressively move from walking with the aid of assistive devices to walking on their own. To help improve healing, physical therapy sessions may also start to emphasize strengthening exercises and functional tasks.

With the approval of your healthcare physician, you can begin to resume more demanding activities, such as driving and light exercise, after three months. Even though it may take up to six months or more to fully heal, hitting this milestone shows how committed you are to the rehabilitation process and how closely you followed the post-operative care guidelines.

It's critical to keep in mind that mending is a process that takes time and that pushing yourself too hard or anticipating instant results will impede your development. Restored mobility and freedom from bunion pain are goals that can be attained with time and patience, so celebrate every small victory along the road.

The Value Of Confirmation Meetings

Following bunion surgery, follow-up appointments are a crucial component of the post-operative treatment regimen. Even while it could be tempting to ignore or put off these visits, doing so raises the possibility of problems and could negatively affect your long-term results. A complete recovery depends on committing to regular appointments and realizing the significance of follow-up care.

Your healthcare professional will evaluate your recovery, track your progress, and handle any issues or difficulties that may come up during follow-up visits. During these sessions, your recovery trajectory can be monitored, any necessary modifications to your treatment plan can be made, and advice on resuming regular activities can be given.

Follow-up visits enable a comprehensive assessment of functional results and overall satisfaction with the surgical outcome, in addition to assessing physical healing. Your doctor will ask you about your pain threshold, range of motion, and capacity for carrying out daily tasks to gain important insight into the status of your recuperation.

Follow-up visits are essential for long-term monitoring and preventive treatment, even after the initial post-operative phase. Frequent check-ups minimize the chance of complications and improve long-term results by enabling your healthcare professional to spot and manage any possible problems early.

In conclusion, follow-up visits are an essential part of thorough post-operative treatment and not merely a formality. You may get the most out of bunion surgery and continue to benefit from better foot health and mobility for years to come if you show up for these appointments on time and work hard during your rehabilitation.

Exercises For Physical Therapy And Rehabilitation

Following bunion surgery, physical therapy and rehabilitation activities are crucial parts of the healing process. These exercises are essential for maximizing results and lowering the chance of problems because they are made to restore strength, flexibility, and function to the injured foot.

Your physical therapy program will be customized to meet your specific needs and may involve a mix of exercises for proprioception, balance, strength, and stretching.

By focusing on particular muscles and joints used in walking and weight-bearing, these exercises serve to enhance stability, range of motion, and general foot mechanics.

Physical therapy's initial goals during the healing process are to lessen discomfort and swelling, encourage healing, and avoid stiffness.

To move the big toe joint and surrounding tissues, gentle range-of-motion exercises and manual treatments can be employed, which can enhance circulation and promote tissue repair.

As you move through the healing process, functional mobility and strength restoration become the main goals of physical therapy. Exercises involving weight bearing, such as toe raises and heel raises, improve balance and stability when walking and performing other weight-bearing tasks by strengthening the muscles of the foot and ankle.

Exercises for balance and proprioception are also crucial parts of rehabilitation since they enhance coordination and lower the chance of falls. To stress the neuromuscular system, these workouts could involve standing on one leg, utilizing stability discs or balancing boards, and engaging in dynamic motions.

After bunion surgery, consistency and devotion to your physical therapy program are essential for getting the best results.

Through active participation in treatment sessions and following exercise regimens at home, you can decrease discomfort and stiffness, expedite the healing process, and restore your confidence in your capacity to move with ease and efficiency.

Modifying Everyday Tasks While Recovering

To maximize results after bunion surgery to promote healing and minimize discomfort, everyday activities must be modified throughout the recovery period. While it's reasonable to want to get back to your regular activities as soon as possible, pushing yourself too far or partaking in physically demanding or high-impact activities might hinder your recovery and raise the possibility of issues.

Rest and elevation should be given top priority in the early postoperative phase to minimize swelling and accelerate recovery. To prevent unnecessary stress on the surgical site, limit weight-bearing activities on the affected foot and avoid standing or walking for extended periods.

Reintroduce light everyday responsibilities like cleaning, cooking, and self-care as soon as the discomfort and swelling go away. Utilize assistive technology, such as walkers or crutches, as required to promote movement and lessen pressure on the affected foot.

Pay attention to your body's cues and honor them. Reduce or alter your activity if it causes pain or discomfort to prevent aggravating symptoms. To reduce stress on the foot and encourage healing, concentrate on keeping good posture, employing appropriate body mechanics, and distributing weight evenly.

Under the supervision of your healthcare professional, progressively increase the duration and intensity of your activities as you move through the recovery process. Throughout your everyday routine, incorporate mild stretching and strengthening activities to enhance your flexibility, stability, and functional mobility.

Above all, practice self-compassion and give yourself enough time to relax and heal. Resuming full activity too soon can impede healing and raise the possibility of problems. You may promote a seamless and effective recovery following bunion surgery by paying attention to your body, taking it slow, and making self-care a priority.

Keeping Bunions From Recurring

A vital component of maintaining long-term foot health and general well-being is preventing bunions from recurring. Although surgery for bunions can treat the deformity and relieve discomfort, treating the underlying causes of the condition is crucial to preventing future recurrence.

Wearing the wrong shoes is one of the main causes of bunions. Bunions can be more likely to occur and existing deformities can be made worse by wearing tight, narrow shoes with pointed toes. To save undue strain on the big toe joint and to suit the natural contours of your foot, look for shoes with a broad toe box and sufficient arch support.

Recurrence of bunions can also be avoided by eating a balanced, nutrient-rich diet and staying at a healthy weight.

Being overweight puts additional strain on the feet and may be a factor in structural deformities that increase the risk of developing bunions. Aim for a healthy weight by combining mindful eating with frequent activity.

Bunions are mostly caused by biomechanical anomalies and foot mechanics. Correcting biomechanical anomalies and lowering the chance of bunion recurrence can be achieved by addressing underlying gait problems, muscle imbalances, and joint dysfunction with the assistance of a podiatrist or physical therapist.

Ultimately, you can protect yourself against the recurrence of bunions by implementing preventive measures into your everyday routine.

Maintaining the health of your feet and lowering the risk of future issues can be accomplished with regular foot care, appropriate footwear selection, and stretching and strengthening exercises.

By taking a comprehensive approach to foot care and treating the underlying causes of bunions as well as their symptoms, you can reduce the likelihood of a recurrence and benefit from improved foot health and mobility for years to come.

CHAPTER SIX

COMMON ISSUES AND DIFFICULTIES

Similar to any surgical operation, bunion surgery is not without its dangers and potential complications. To guarantee that the healing process goes well, it is essential to be aware of these in advance. The possibility of infection is one frequent worry. Post-operative infections are possible, however uncommon. However, this danger is considerably lower if you adhere to the wound care guidelines prescribed by your healthcare practitioner.

The potential for blood clots to form in the legs following surgery is another issue. Those who are elderly or suffer from specific medical issues are more in danger. Your surgeon might advise using compression stockings and doing easy leg exercises while you heal to lessen this risk.

Following bunion surgery, complications include stiffness and restricted range of motion in the toe joint are also possible. Your healthcare professional can recommend physical therapy and exercises to address this transient condition. Recurrence of the bunion is another possible consequence. Although the deformity is intended to be corrected by surgery, there is a slight possibility that the bunion will eventually recur. However, this risk can be reduced by adhering to post-surgery instructions, such as donning orthotics and supportive footwear.

Handling Pain And Discomfort After Surgery

After bunion surgery, controlling pain and discomfort is an essential part of the healing process. Pain medication will be prescribed by your healthcare professional to help ease any discomfort you may be feeling. It's critical to take these drugs as prescribed and to avoid delaying taking them until the pain gets really bad. Furthermore, using cold packs on the surgery site can help numb the region and minimize swelling, which will ease pain.

Reducing swelling and pain can also be achieved by raising your foot above your heart. You can achieve this by sleeping or relaxing with your foot propped up on pillows. For your body to repair correctly in the early phases of recovery, rest is just as crucial. Take part in activities that involve little movement and refrain from placing weight on the affected foot. To avoid stiffness and increase circulation, it's crucial to find a balance between rest and light exercise.

Handling Bruises And Swelling

After bunion surgery, swelling and bruises are frequent side effects that can be easily treated with appropriate treatment. Short bursts of ice packs applied to the surgery site can help minimize pain and edema. To avoid direct skin contact with the ice pack, which can result in ice burns, it is imperative to wrap it in a cloth or towel. By encouraging the outflow of extra fluid, raising your foot above your heart level can also aid in the reduction of edema.

Additionally, reducing swelling and enhancing blood circulation in the injured foot can be achieved by donning compression stockings or socks. By encouraging lymphatic drainage, a little massage around the surgical site can also help lessen bruising and swelling. To be sure a massage is safe for your particular condition, you should always speak with your doctor before attempting any new techniques.

Preventing Infections And Recognizing Warning Signs

After bunion surgery, preventing infection is essential to a full recovery. You will receive detailed instructions from your healthcare practitioner on how to take care of the surgical site to reduce the chance of infection. This usually entails changing dressings as directed, keeping the wound dry and clean, and avoiding submerging the foot in water. To lower the possibility of problems, it is imperative that you carefully follow these directions.

Increased warmth, redness, or swelling around the surgical site, together with pus or drainage from the wound, are warning signs of infection. For more assessment and treatment, you must get in touch with your healthcare professional right away if you encounter any of these symptoms. Timely medical intervention is vital as the illness may require antibiotics in certain circumstances.

Taking Care Of Cosmetic Concerns And Scarring

After bunion surgery, scarring is a normal part of the healing process, but there are things you can do to lessen how noticeable it is. Reducing the likelihood of severe scarring and promoting healthy healing can be achieved by keeping the surgery site hydrated and clean. Additionally, to help break down scar tissue and enhance the appearance of the scar, your healthcare expert could suggest scar massage procedures.

Talk to your healthcare professional if you have any specific cosmetic concerns about the scar's appearance, such as its size or visibility. Scar revision surgery is a possible option in certain circumstances to make the scar look better. However, before thinking about any further operations, it is imperative to wait until the surgical site has healed completely.

Taking Care Of Nerve Damage And Mobility Problems

Following bunion surgery, nerve damage and mobility problems are possible, but they are often transient and become better with time with the right treatment and therapy. Physical therapy activities may be recommended by your healthcare physician to assist the injured foot regain its strength and range of motion. To avoid stiffness and encourage healing, these exercises must be performed regularly.

In addition, orthotics and supportive footwear can aid in stabilizing and supporting the foot as it heals. It's critical to let your healthcare professional know if you continue to feel numb or tingly in the afflicted foot. They can assess your symptoms and suggest the best course of action, including medication or additional testing by a specialist.

Nerve damage and movement problems can be properly controlled with the right care and attention, allowing you to resume your regular activities with the least amount of inconvenience.

CHAPTER SEVEN

COMMONLY ASKED QUESTIONS OR FAQS

Since bunion surgery can be a big decision, it makes sense that patients would have a lot of concerns regarding the process, possible outcomes, and recuperation. These are a few typical questions:

How Likely Is It That Bunions Will Recur?

After surgery, bunions may reoccur, however this is not very common. The degree of the bunion, the kind of surgery done, and the post-operative care all have a significant role in how well the procedure goes. In general, recurrence risk has been considerably lower with modern surgical techniques than with traditional approaches. To reduce the likelihood of a recurrence, you must strictly adhere to your surgeon's post-operative orders. Frequently, these guidelines involve donning supportive footwear, steering clear of strenuous activities, and keeping follow-up appointments to receive monitoring.

How Soon After Surgery Can I Go On Foot?

The amount of time it takes to walk following bunion surgery varies based on the type of procedure and personal characteristics like healing capacity and general health. To reduce stiffness and improve blood circulation, patients are frequently advised to begin walking with the use of crutches or a walker soon after surgery. But initially, you might not be able to bear much weight, and you might need to increase your activity level gradually over a few weeks. To guarantee a secure and effective recovery, your surgeon will offer you particular instructions based on your circumstances.

Will I Require Certain Shoes After My Surgery?

Yes, it is very important to wear proper shoes during the healing phase after bunion surgery. Your physician could suggest certain shoe styles that provide your toes plenty of space and sufficient foot support. To help maintain correct alignment and stop recurrence, tailored orthotic inserts may also be prescribed in specific circumstances. Shoes that are too tight or thin must be avoided as they may worsen the development of bunions or apply pressure on the surgery site. To guarantee the best possible comfort and recuperation, make sure you and your surgeon talk about your footwear options.

Can I Lose My Ability To Exercise After Bunion Surgery?

Your ability to participate in some physical activities, especially those that require high-impact or repeated movements that could strain the foot, may be temporarily restricted following bunion surgery. But if your surgeon gives the all-clear and you've healed completely, you ought to be able to gradually go back into your workout regimen. During the early phases of recuperation, low-impact exercises like yoga, cycling, and swimming are frequently advised to preserve cardiovascular health and flexibility without putting undue strain on the feet. You can progressively return to more strenuous activities as you advance, but be careful to listen to your body and refrain from overdoing it.

What Kind Of Lifestyle Adjustments Are Required After Surgery?

Making specific lifestyle adjustments after bunion surgery can greatly speed up healing and reduce the chance of recurrence. These could consist of:

Foot care involves taking proper care of your feet and checking them frequently for symptoms of infection or other problems.

Good Practices: Refraining from smoking, which can slow recovery and raise the risk of problems, eating a balanced diet, and drinking plenty of water.

Physical therapy: Performing stretches and exercises as directed to increase ankle and foot strength, flexibility, and range of motion.

Choosing supportive, well-fitting shoes with a roomy toe box will help to support your foot shape and lessen strain on the surgical site.

Frequent Follow-ups: Keep track of and receive direction from your surgeon during the recovery process by attending planned follow-up sessions.

These lifestyle adjustments can help you get the most out of your bunion surgery and maintain comfortable, healthy feet for years to come.

www.ingramcontent.com/pod-product-compliance
Lightning Source LLC
Chambersburg PA
CBHW071843210526
45479CB00001B/268